A Simple W Cookbook:

Quick and Easy Single Portion Recipes for Lasting Weight Loss

Table of Contents

Table of Contents 2

Introduction 3

Chapter 1: 20 Energizing Breakfast Recipes 6

Chapter 2: 20 Filling Low- Carb Lunch Recipes .. 22

Chapter 3: Dinner for One: 20 Recipes to Cook at Home 42

Chapter 4: 10 Sweet Desserts that Curb Cravings 65

Chapter 5: 10 Crockpot Single and Double Serving Recipes 75

Chapter 6: 25 Meal Replacement Smoothies 85

Conclusion 99

Introduction

Thank you and congratulations on downloading *A Simple Weight Loss Cookbook: Quick and Easy Single Portion Recipes for Lasting Weight Loss*!

We all know the struggle of trying to lose a few pounds. Our year starts with a resolution to drop three pants sizes, climaxes into the dreaded summer months of bathing suit weather and then resolves once again to feelings of regret and remorse as we enjoy yet another helping of mom's Christmas feast. Although many of us wish that we could go to the gym and enjoy only eating salad, the reality is that our busy lives keep us from pursuing a weight loss regiment for more than a few weeks. And once we start getting the results we want, we end up cheating on the program and binge on a sugary, carb- filled meal.

The problem is, there are many issues with dieting programs that you find on the internet or in bookstores. Firstly, these regiments only account for a few weeks or months' worth of meals. This means that after going through the entire meal plan and grocery list three or four times, you are left having to make the same boring recipes again and again in order to keep off the weight you just lost. How many times are you supposed to go through the same cycle before it stops working or you get so tired of the same food that you cheat on your diet?

Secondly, most recipes that are included in weight loss programs make serving sizes big enough to feed a family of four. If you are single, why would you make so much food for just one meal? Or perhaps your partner does not want to participate in this new meal plan and you have to struggle to cut down the recipe measurement? And any parent knows that getting your kids to eat is already a nightly struggle, and trying to force them to taste new foods is a whole other battle.

This cookbook cuts out the common problems that healthy eaters always come across with other programs by providing a variety of easy, single serving recipes for you to enjoy! This book contains recipes that are proven to help you lose weight, save money on groceries, and continue making progress towards your health and fitness goals. The ingredients this book encourages you to use are fresh and provide you with the necessary proteins, fats, and carbohydrates that will fulfill your daily nutritional requirements.

Here is an inescapable fact: everyone wishes that they could lose weight by eating delicious food. While the instructions in this book won't have you carbo- loading on pasta, they will make cooking for yourself easier and much more enjoyable. With over *seventy* recipes included, the meals in this book are delicious and diverse, so you will always have new flavors to try. You no longer have to sacrifice great flavor to achieve that desired pant size. You can achieve your fitness goals and come to love and nourish your body just by following these recipes.

The best part about this weight loss cookbook is that you don't need any fancy kitchen equipment or school taught techniques to make them. With any standard kitchen, you can prepare all of these recipes in less than a half an hour, so you can still satisfy your sweet and savory cravings without worrying about bingeing or cheating during your meals.

It's time for you to become an amazing chef with an even more amazing body! In no time at all, you will finally have the physique of your dreams. Without any special tricks, costly supplements, or advice from a top notch professional trainer you will easily burn fat and becoming a healthier, better you. Thank you again for downloading this book. Good luck on your health and wellness journey; enjoy every last bite!

Chapter 1: 20 Energizing Breakfast Recipes

1. Classic Smoked Salmon on Toast

<u>Ingredients</u>

    2 Oz. of Smoked Salmon

    ½ Tbs. of Chives

    1 Slice of Whole Grain Bread

    1 Slice of Red Onion

    1 Tbs. of Cream Cheese

<u>Directions</u>

1. Simply toast your slice of whole grain bread before adding a thin coat of cream cheese on top.
2. Next, place your fresh salmon cuts over the cream cheese layer, followed by the slice of sweet red onion.
3. Top your decadent breakfast with a sprinkle of chives and enjoy!

Calorie Estimate: 350

2. Ham and Cheese Engnlish Breakfast

<u>Ingredients</u>

    2 Oz of Sliced Black Forest Ham

    2 Tbs. of Light Cheddar Cheese

    1 Whole Wheat English Muffin

    ¼ Cup of Kale, torn with stems removed

    ¼ Cup of Spinach, leaves torn

    1 tsp. of Extra Virgin Olive Oil

Directions

1. Start off by lightly toasting your English muffin halves.
2. Once toasted, begin layering the rest of the solid ingredients onto your muffin halves. Starting with the ham, followed by the greens, then cheese.
3. Next, drizzle the open sandwich with the teaspoon of olive oil.
4. Place the English muffin halves into a preheated oven set at 375 degrees Fahrenheit. Continue toasting the muffin halves until the cheese melts onto the bread.

Calorie Estimate: 300

    3. Sweet Potato Wedges with Sausage

Ingredients

    3 Links of Chicken and Sage Sausage

    1 Sweet Potato, roughly chopped into cubes

    2 Tbs. of Extra Virgin Olive Oil

    1 Cup of Baby Spinach

Directions:

1. Start by heating your oven to 350 degrees. Place your sausage on a baking sheet and transfer into the oven.

2. In a skillet, sauté the sweet potato cubes in olive oil until they become soft. Add in the spinach leaves and stir gently.

3. Once the sausage is heated and cooked all the way through, remove the baking sheet from the oven. Transfer your sausage and vegetables onto a plate.

4. Season with red pepper, pink Himalayan sea salt, or Italian herbs. Enjoy!

Calorie Estimate: 300

4. Breakfast Egg and Veggie Quesadilla

Ingredients

    1 Whole Egg

    1 Egg White

    1 8-in. Whole Wheat Tortilla

    ¼ White Onion, diced

    ¼ Red Pepper, Diced

    1 Oz. of Mozzarella Cheese

    2 Tbs. of Salsa

Directions

1. Start by heating your pepper and onion in a heated skillet. When the vegetables are almost fully cooked, pour in the whisked eggs and scramble the ingredients together.

2. Once the ingredients are mixed together in the pan, fold the eggs into the tortilla and top with cheese. Fold the tortilla to make a breakfast quesadilla.

3. Simply pour the salsa over top of your quesadilla or cut the tortilla into slices to dip into the salsa.

Calorie Estimate: 330

5. Ricotta and Honey Breakfast for Sweet Tooth's

Ingredients

- 1 Cup of Part-Skim Ricotta Cheese
- ½ Cup of Mango, chopped
- 1 tsp. of Organic Honey
- ½ Tbs. of Ground Flaxseed

Directions

1. Simply scoop the ricotta cheese into a small bowl. Next, drizzle in the honey and stir in the flaxseeds.
2. Finally, top your sweet breakfast with the mango and enjoy!

Calorie Estimate: 400

6. Cottage Cheese and Egg Muffin Breakfast

Ingredients

- 1 Whole Wheat English Muffin
- 1 Hard Boiled Egg
- ½ Cup of Light Cottage Cheese
- 2 Strawberries, sliced

Directions

1. Start out your breakfast by toasting your English muffin halves. As your muffin is heating up, peel your hardboiled egg and slice it. Top your toasted muffin halves with the slices of egg.

2. Complete your breakfast by simply mixing the cottage cheese with the strawberries. Keep in mind that you can enjoy many different fruits with cottage cheese, so you can mix up this recipe a dozen different ways!

Calorie Estimate: 350

7. Artichoke and Tomato Protein Frittata

<u>Ingredients</u>

1 Whole Egg

1 Egg White

½ Tomato, Diced

2 Tbs. of Feta Cheese, crumbled

1.2 Cup of Canned Artichoke Hearts, drained and diced

<u>Directions</u>

1. Start by whisking your egg and egg white together. Heat a skillet to medium heat and coat with cooking spray.

2. Add the tomato and artichoke to the pan and cook for about two minutes.

3. Reduce the heat to a lower setting before slowly pouring the eggs into pan.

4. Cover your skillet and let the ingredients cook for approximately three minutes, until the eggs are cooked and firm.

5. Remove the frittata from the skillet and top with the crumbled feta cheese. Enjoy!

Calorie Estimate: 250

8. Yogurt and Fruit Parfait

<u>Ingredients</u>

8 Oz. of Light Greek Yogurt

½ tsp. of Organic Honey

½ Medium Grapefruit

1 tsp. of Ground Flaxseed

<u>Directions</u>

1. Start by combining the flaxseed and yogurt.
2. In a tall cup, stack alternating layers of the grapefruit and yogurt until you reach the rim of the glass.
3. Drizzle on some sweet honey and enjoy!

Calorie Estimate: 250

9. Pumpkin Pancakes

<u>Ingredients</u>

½ Cup of Pumpkin Puree

1 Egg

2 Tbs. of Almond Flour

¼ tsp. of Allspice

¼ tsp. of Pumpkin Spice

¼ tsp. of Cinnamon

Directions

1. Start by beating the egg in a small bowl. Next, mix in the pumpkin puree until well- combined.

2. Once you have mixed together the egg and pumpkin, add in the almond flour and combine into the other ingredients.

3. Heat your skillet over medium- high heat and lightly coat with cooking spray. Spoon one tablespoon of your pancake batter onto the skillet to form each pancake. Cook each pancake until the batter begins to form bubbles and the edges become firm.

4. Gently flip the pancakes and allow the underside to cook. When both sides are cooked and a light golden brown, remove the pancakes from the skillet onto a plate.

5. Enjoy with a half a tablespoon of light maple syrup or honey!

Calorie Estimate: 210

10. Nut Butter and Strawberry Breakfast Wrap

Ingredients

2 Tbs. of Almond Butter

1 8-in. Whole Wheat Tortilla

½ Cup of Sliced Strawberries

Directions

1. Simply spread the almond butter evenly onto the tortilla. Next, layer on the strawberry slices.

2. Roll up the tortilla and enjoy with a cup of chilled almond milk!

Calorie Estimate: 370

11. Citrus Fruit Salad

Ingredients

1 Red Grapefruit

1 Navel Orange

¼ of a Lime

½ Cup of Blueberries

Directions

1. Start by cutting the peel and white pith from the orange and grapefruit. Then, cut the orange and grapefruit into pieces, placing them into a small bowl.

2. Next, squeeze the lime wedge over top of the fruit. Finish your fruit salad by carefully tossing the blueberries into the mix. Enjoy!

Calorie Estimate: 220

12. Low- Carb Banana Pancakes

Ingredients

1 Large Extra Ripe Banana

2 Large Eggs

¼ Cup of Almond Butter

Directions

1. Start by peeling the banana, then mashing it with a fork in a medium- size bowl.

2. Add in the almond butter and continue mashing the banana and nut butter until you achieve a smooth consistency. Next, add in the eggs and whisk them with a fork. Continue combining the mixture until the ingredients are incorporated into a blended batter.

3. Heat a skillet over medium- low heat and lightly coat with cooking spray. Spoon two tablespoons of batter into the skillet to create one pancake. Cook the pancake on one side until bubble begin to form and disperse and the edges of the cake become firm.

4. Flip the pancake and continue cooking on the other side for one more minute until the underside becomes golden brown.

5. Enjoy your low- carb pancakes with half a tablespoon of honey or a glass of chilled almond milk.

Calorie Estimate: 450

13. Toasted Coconut Oatmeal

<u>Ingredients</u>

1 Serving of Quick- Cooking Rolled Oats

2 Tbs. of Coconut Flakes, unsweetened

1 Tbs. of Cashews, roughly chopped

2 tsp. of Brown Sugar

¼ Cup of Mango, chopped

<u>Directions</u>

1. Preheat your oven to 350 degrees. Prepare a baking sheet with aluminum foil. Start by spreading the coconut across the baking sheet. Toast in the oven for three to five minutes, until they achieve a golden tone.

2. Prepare your serving of oats in accordance with the provided instructions on the packaging. Once you have cooked the oats, sprinkle the brown sugar on top and mix into the oatmeal.

3. Finally, top your oatmeal with the coconut, mango, and cashews.

Calorie Estimate: 250

14. Sunflower and Blueberry Oatmeal

Ingredients

1 Serving of Quick-Cookie Rolled Oats

1 Tbs. of Unshelled Sunflower Seeds

½ Cup of Blueberries

½ Tbs. of Honey

Directions

1. Simply prepare your oats according to the instructions provided on the packaging.

2. Top off your oatmeal with the fruit and seeds before drizzling the honey on top. Enjoy!

Calorie Estimate: 200

15. Savory Egg and Avocado Oatmeal

Ingredients

1 Serving of Quick- Cooking Rolled Oats

1 Large Egg

¼ of an Avocado, sliced

2 tsp. of Extra Virgin Olive Oil

1 Tbs. of Salsa

Directions

1. Start by preparing your oats according to the instructions provided on the packaging.
2. As the oats are cooking, heat the olive oil in a skillet over medium heat. Crack your egg into the skillet and cook sunny-side up. Simply do this by cracking the egg into the pan, then covering it for two to four minutes until the egg whites have become solid while the yolk remains liquid on the inside.
3. Transfer your egg from the pan to the top of your oatmeal. Add in the sliced avocado and salsa, and enjoy!

Calorie Estimate: 200

16. Vanilla and Almond Chia Seed Pudding

Ingredients

½ Cup of Vanilla Flavored Almond Milk

¼ tsp. of Ground Cinnamon

2 ½ Tbs. of Chia Seeds

1 Pinch of Pink Himalayan Sea Salt

½ Tbs. of Agave Nectar

¼ tsp. of Vanilla Extract

Directions

1. This is a recipe that requires a bit more preparation time than usual. It will take approximately two hours for the chia seeds to absorb the almond milk. Therefore, you should prepare your breakfast first thing in the morning before starting your morning routine.

2. Start by combining all of the ingredients in a large bowl. Stir together the ingredients until well combined. Make sure that the seeds are entirely coated in the almond milk.

3. Cover the bowl with aluminum foil and place in the refrigerator. Refrigerate for approximately two hours. When the pudding is thick, remove from the refrigerator and stir. Enjoy!

Calorie Estimate: 200

17. Stuffed Tomatoes

Ingredients

1 Large Garden Tomato

1 Large Egg

¼ Cup of Shredded Light Cheddar Cheese

½ an Onion, chopped

1 tsp. of Extra Virgin Olive Oil

1 tsp. of Ginger- Garlic Paste

A Pinch of Dried Parsley

Directions:

1. Start by thoroughly washing your tomato. Then, cut the top and bottom off of the tomato, so that it can stand up straight. Use a spoon to scoop out the flesh of the tomato, ensuring that the shell is still intact. Your tomato should look like a small bowl.

2. In a skillet, head up the olive oil and fry your onion and ginger- garlic paste. Add in the parsley and allow the vegetables to cook. Then, remove from the pan and allow to cool.

3. Prepare a baking sheet with aluminum foil and place your tomato onto the sheet. Preheat your oven to 180 degrees Fahrenheit.

4. Spoon the onion mixture into the tomato, so that it is filled halfway. Next, crack your egg into the tomato bowl.

5. Top your egg with the cheddar cheese and then place in the oven for approximately twelve to fifteen minutes, or until the tomato skin starts to wrinkle.

Calorie Estimate: 180

18. Breakfast Skillet Stir-fry

Ingredients

1 cup of Frozen Shredded Hash Brown Potatoes

¼ Cup of Shredded Light Cheddar Cheese

1 Large Egg

1 Slice of Bacon, cooked and chopped

¼ Tbs. of Extra Virgin Olive Oil

Directions

1. Heat a small skillet over medium heat and add in the olive oil.
2. Once the oil is hot, place the potatoes into the pan and allow to cook until the potatoes become brown and crisp. Season with salt, pepper, and red pepper if desired.
3. While your potatoes are cooking, crack the egg into a bowl and whisk to scramble. Preheat your oven to 350 degrees.
4. Next, add the eggs, bacon, and cheese into the small pan with the potatoes. Scramble the ingredients together to make a stir- fry. Do not cook the eggs all the way through.
5. Remove the skillet from the stovetop and carefully place in the oven for approximately five minutes, or until the eggs have set and the cheese is melted. Enjoy!

Calorie Estimate: 460

19. Kate's Fresh Garden Stir-fry

Ingredients

    1 Large Egg

    1 Egg White

    ¼ of a Red Bell Pepper, diced

    ½ a Tomato, Diced

    ¼ Cup of Crumbled Feta Cheese

    ¼ tsp. of Dried Mixed Herbs

    1 Slice of Whole Grain Bread

2 tsp. of Extra Virgin Olive Oil

Directions

1. Start by heating a skillet over medium heat, adding in the olive oil as the pan heats up.

2. Once the oil is hot, add in the diced tomato and red bell pepper to the pan. Stir the contents of the pan occasionally and cook until the vegetables are almost cooked through.

3. As the vegetables are heating up, crack the egg into a small bowl and whisk. Place the slice of whole- grain into the toaster and lightly toast.

4. Add the egg into the pan and scramble into the vegetables until the eggs are almost thoroughly cooked. Then, add in the feta cheese and fold into the egg-vegetable mixture until the cheese has melted.

5. Remove the bread from the toaster. Scoop the contents of the skillet onto the piece of toast, and top with the dried herbs. Enjoy!

Calorie Estimate: 280

20. Low- Carb Blueberry Pancakes

Ingredients

½ Cup of Old- Fashioned Rolled Oats

½ Cup of Blueberries

¼ of a Cup of Low- Fat Cottage Cheese

1 Egg

½ tsp. of Vanilla Extract

Directions

1. Start by combining your oats, egg, cottage cheese, and vanilla extract in a blender or food processor. Pulse the ingredients until you achieve a smooth consistency. Next, add in the blueberries. Do not blend into the batter, but simply fold into the oats.

2. Heat a skillet over medium heat and prepare with a coating of cooking spray. Spoon two tablespoons of the batter onto the pan to create one pancake. Cook the cake for approximately three minutes, until bubbles begin to appear on the top and the edges are cooked. Then, flip the pancake and continue cooking until the underside is golden brown.

3. Remove from heat and enjoy with a side of low- yogurt.

Chapter 2: 20 Filling Low- Carb Lunch Recipes

1. Cauliflower and Shrimp Salad

<u>Ingredients</u>

¼ Head of Cauliflower

¼ lb. of Raw Shrimp

½ Tbs. of Extra Virgin Olive Oil

½ a Cucumber

1 Tbs. of Lemon Juice

1 tsp. of Lemon Zest

<u>Directions</u>

1. Start by peeling, cleaning, and removing the tails of your shrimp.
2. Preheat your oven to 350 degrees and prepare a baking sheet with cooking spray or aluminum foil. Place your shrimp onto the sheet and drizzle half a tablespoon of olive oil on top. Add seasoning if desired. Place the baking sheet in the oven and cook for eight to ten minutes, or until they become opaque.
3. As the shrimp is cooking, cut off the cauliflower florets, tossing away the bottom stalk. Cut the cauliflower into small pieces, so they will be easier to break down later. Next, place the cauliflower to in a microwave- safe dish and microwave for approximately four to five minutes. Make sure that it cooks evenly and becomes soft, but not mushy in texture.

4. When the cauliflower and shrimp are cooling, begin to seed, peel, and chop the cucumber into small ½ in. pieces.
5. Once your shrimp have cooled down enough to handle, slice them into halves. In a medium bowl, combine your ingredients, adding the lemon juice and zest on top of your salad.

Calorie Estimate: 210

2. Zucchini Pasta with Tomato Basil Sauce

<u>Ingredients</u>

- ½ Cup of Cherry Tomatoes
- 2 Tbs. of Oil Packed Sun-Dried Tomatoes
- 1 Single Serving of Angel Hair Pasta
- 1 Large Poached Egg
- 1 Oz. of Grated Parmesan Cheese
- 1 Tbs. of Minced Kalamata Olives
- 1 Tbs. of Extra Virgin Olive Oil
- ¼ Cup of Fresh Basil, roughly chopped
- ½ Tbs. of Toasted Pine Nuts
- ½ Tbs. of Minced Garlic
- 1 Lemon Wedge
- 1 Medium Zucchini

<u>Directions</u>

1. Start by bringing a small pot of salted water to a boil. While you water comes to a boil, finely chop half of your cherry tomatoes and place them in a bowl.

2. Add in the sun- dried tomatoes to the bowl, with the basil, garlic, and squeeze the juice from the lemon wedge into the mixture as well. Season with salt and pepper if desired. Set aside and let sit for at least five minutes.

3. When the water starts boiling, add in the pasta and cook according to the instructions provided on the packaging. Then drain and set aside.

4. While the pasta is cooking, use a spiralizer to transform the solid zucchini into long spirals of noodles. Add the zucchini noodles into the bowl with the hot spaghetti noodles and allow the heat to slightly cook the vegetable noodles. Add in the olives and olive oil and toss the mixture well.

5. Add the tomato sauce onto the pasta, topped with the poached egg. Break the poached egg and toss in the pasta to create a thicker sauce. Top with the parmesan cheese and basil. Enjoy!

Calorie Estimate: 580

3. Low- Carb Mushroom Burger

Ingredients

      1 Tbs. of Extra Virgin Olive Oil

      1 ½ Tbs. of Balsamic Vinegar

      2 Portabella Mushroom Caps, stems removed

      1 Slice of Halloumi Cheese

      1 Slice of Tomato

Directions

1. Preheat your grill to medium- high heat, approximately 450 degrees.

2. Wash the mushroom caps and gently dry. Then, in a small bowl, combine the vinegar and olive oil. Dip the mushrooms into the oil and vinegar mixture, gill side down.

3. Place the mushrooms onto the heated grill and allow to cook for five minutes, until they begin to seat. Then, flip the mushrooms over and grill for another three minutes.

4. Place the halloumi on the grill and cook on either side for two minutes until the cheese becomes soft and pliable.

5. Create your 'burger' by using the mushroom as the bun, the cheese as the burger patty, and then top with the tomato and basil for added flavor.

Calorie Estimate: 330

4. Spaghetti Squash Lunch

Ingredients

1 Spaghetti Squash

1 Clove of Garlic

1 Tbs. of Extra Virgin Olive Oil

½ Cup of Kale Leaves, stems removed

½ Can of Cooked Chickpeas

1 Oz. of Grated Parmesan Cheese

Directions:

1. Preheat your oven to 400 degrees and prepare a baking sheet with cooking spray or aluminum foil.

2. Begin this recipe by cutting the spaghetti squash in half, lengthwise. Then, remove the seeds and rub the inside of both halves with half of the olive oil. Next, place the squash facing down onto the baking sheet. Place into the oven for forty- five minutes.

3. As the squash is baking, wash the kale leaves before roughly chopping them into small pieces.

4. In a skillet, heat the last half- tablespoon of olive oil and cook the garlic and kale until the leaves turn a vibrant green. Add in the chickpeas and cook to warm them.

5. Remove both the squash and chickpea- kale mixture from heat. Use a fork to scrape out the inside of the squash halves. The flesh will pull away from the shell in a similar shape to spaghetti.

6. Put the strands of cooked squash into a bowl and toss with the kale mixture. Serve the squash and kale salad in a bowl or right from the spaghetti squash shells. Sprinkle the parmesan cheese on top and enjoy!

Calorie Estimate: 230

5. Chicken and Asparagus Stir Fry

Ingredients

2 Thin Boneless, Skinless Chicken Breasts, cut into 1- in. cubes

3 Tbs. of Low- Sodium Chicken Broth

½ Tbs. of Low- Sodium Soy Sauce

½ tsp. of Cornstarch

½ Tbs. of Water

¼ Tbs. of Grapeseed Oil

½ Bunch of Asparagus, ends trimmed and stalks cut into 2- in. pieces

2 Cloves of Garlic Chopped, chopped

2 tsp. of Fresh Ginger

½ Tbs. of Fresh Lemon Juice

Directions

1. Season your chicken with salt and pepper. In a small bowl, mix together the soy sauce and broth. In a separate bowl, combine the water and cornstarch until the ingredients are completely incorporated together.

2. Preheat a skillet over medium- high heat. Add the grapeseed oil into the pan and fry the asparagus until the stalks become tender and crispy. Add the garlic and ginger into the pan as well and cook until they become golden brown. Set the mixture aside when you are finished cooking.

3. Increase the heat to a higher setting and use a separate pan to cook the chicken in another teaspoon or so of grapeseed oil. Cook the chicken until it is cooked through and browned. Then, remove from heat and set aside.

4. Next, bring the soy sauce mixture to a boil and let cook for approximately one minute. Then, add in the lemon juice and cornstarch mix: stir together well. Toss the chicken and asparagus together. When the soy sauce begins to simmer, drizzle over the chicken and asparagus. Enjoy!

Calorie Estimate: 260

6. Chickpea and Salmon Salad

<u>Ingredients</u>

- 1 Can of Salmon, drained
- ½ Can of Chickpeas, rinsed and drained
- ½ Stalk of Celery, sliced thin
- 1 Shallot, minced
- ½ Clove of Garlic, minced
- ½ Red Bell Pepper, sliced thin
- ¼ of a Cucumber, chopped
- ½ Cup of Cherry Tomatoes, sliced in half
- 2 Tbs. of Extra Virgin Olive Oil
- 2 tsp. of Red Wine Vinegar

<u>Directions</u>

1. Pour the chickpeas into a medium- size bowl. Finely chop and mince your celery, pepper, tomatoes, cucumber, and shallots: add the ingredients into the bowl with the chickpeas.
2. Drain the salmon if you haven't already, and then add the fish into the bowl. Season the dish as you see fit, then allow the salad to sit in the refrigerator for at least one hour.

Calorie Estimate: 330

7. Vegetable Sushi- Inspired Rolls

<u>Ingredients</u>

- 2 Raw Sushi Nori Sheets
- 1 Carrot, cut into thin strips
- 1 Avocado
- ¼ of a Zucchini, cut into thin strips
- ½ Red Bell Pepper, sliced thin
- ½ Cup of Alfalfa Sprouts

<u>Directions</u>

1. Place your nori sheets onto a flat counter top or cutting board. Then, slice the avocado in half, remove the pit, and mash the inside into a small bowl.
2. Spread half of the avocado onto one side of the nori sheet.
3. Next, strategically horizontally lay the bell pepper slices, carrots, and zucchini onto the nori sheets on top of the mashed avocado. Top off the spread with the sprouts.
4. Quickly but carefully roll the edge of the nori sheet until you can no longer see the filling, rolling until the entire sheet is rolled up. Use water to wet your index finger, and then use the moisture to dampen the nori sheet. Press the edge of the sheet into the roll, so that it become sealed.
5. Repeat this process with the second nori sheet. Slice the rolls into smaller pieces with a knife and enjoy!

Calorie Estimate: 140

8. Shakshuka

<u>Ingredients</u>

    3 tsp. of Extra Virgin Olive Oil

    ¼ of a White Onion, diced

    ½ Clove of Garlic, minced

    ¼ of a Green Bell Pepper, chopped

    ½ Cup of Diced Tomatoes

    ½ Tbs. of Tomato Paste

    2 Eggs

<u>Directions</u>

1. Start by heating up a skillet over medium heat. Slowly warm the oil in the skillet, and add in the diced onions. Sauté the onion until it begins to soften. Add in the garlic and continue to cook until you can smell the garlic becoming fragrant.

2. Next, add in in the green bell pepper and continue sautéing the mixture for another six minutes until the pepper becomes soft. Place the tomatoes and tomato paste into the skillet and stir until blended. Season with salt, pepper, cayenne pepper, and other flavors you enjoy.

3. Reduce the mixture to a simmer and crack each egg, one at a time, into the skillet. Cover the pan and let simmer for ten to fifteen minutes, until the eggs cook. Enjoy with pita bread as a side.

Calorie Estimate: 300

9. Strawberry and Goat Cheese Salad

Ingredients

- ¾ Cup of Grated Goat Cheese
- 2 Cups of Fresh Spinach
- 4 Strawberries, sliced
- ¼ Cup of Toasted Flakes Almonds
- 1 ½ Tbs. of Raspberry Vinaigrette Dressing

Directions

1. Preheat your oven to 400 degrees and prepare a baking sheet with parchment paper. Start your salad by preparing your cheese bowl. Grate your goat cheese onto the baking sheet, letting the shreds fall to create a rough circle.

2. Place the baking sheet into the oven and bake your cheese for approximately ten minutes. It is important to watch the cheese carefully, removing the sheet from the oven when the cheese turns a light gold color. If you bake the cheese for too long, it will become bitter.

3. Remove the cheese from the oven and allow to cool for approximately one minute. Create the cheese bowl by turning a small bowl upside- down, then carefully lift the parchment paper off the of sheet and flip the circle of cooked cheese over the top of the bowl.

4. Lightly press the edges of the cheese to the bowl and let sit for approximately five minutes.

5. Rinse the spinach and then pay dry with a paper towel. Place the spinach into the cheese bowl. Toss in the berry vinaigrette, almonds, and strawberries.

Calorie Estimate: 180

10. Classic Chicken Quesadilla

<u>Ingredients</u>

    3 Oz. of Pepper Jack Cheese

    1 8- in. Whole Wheat Tortilla

    2 Oz. of Grilled Chicken Breast

    1 tsp. Diced Jalapeno Pepper

    2 Tbs. of Chunky Salsa

<u>Directions</u>

1. Start by placing the tortilla wrap onto you're a frying pan over medium heat. Flip the tortilla over after approximately two minutes.
2. Start layering on the pepper jack cheese. Place the grilled chicken breast and jalapeno peppers onto one half of the wrap. Next, fold the tortilla over itself with a spatula, pressing down on it so that the melted cheese acts as a glue to keep it together.
3. Enjoy with the side of chunky salsa!

Calorie Estimate: 550

11. Spinach Cakes

<u>Ingredients</u>

    6 Oz. of Fresh Spinach Leaves

    ¼ Cup of Part-Skim Ricotta Cheese

    ¼ Cup of Shredded Parmesan Cheese

    1 Egg, beaten

½ Clove of Garlic, minced

Directions

1. Preheat your oven to 400 degrees and prepare a muffin pan with cooking spray.
2. Pulse the spinach in two batches to ensure that the leaves become finely chopped. Then, transfer the spinach into a medium bowl and combine with the ricotta cheese, parmesan cheese, egg, and your choice of seasonings.
3. Divide the spinach into four cups of the baking tray. Cake the spinach cakes in the oven until they set; this may take approximately twenty minutes.
4. Remove from the oven and let stand for five minutes. Remove each cake by loosening the edges with a knife. Enjoy with an extra sprinkle of parmesan cheese.

Calorie Estimate: 150/ 2 cakes

12. Eggplant Parmesan

Ingredients

1 Eggplant

1 Egg

3 Oz. of Grated Parmesan Cheesc

1 Clove of Garlic, finely chopped

1 Tbs. of Extra Virgin Olive Oil

Directions

1. Cut the eggplant in half lengthwise and season with salt. Let the eggplant halves sit out for approximately forty-

five minutes. Then, rinse the halves under cold water and use a paper towel to pat dry.

2. Whisk the egg in a deep dish and the parmesan cheese and garlic in a separate dish.

3. Heat the olive oil in a skillet over medium high heat. Dip the eggplant slices into the egg mixture and then into the parmesan cheese mixture as a coating.

4. Lay each eggplant slice onto the skillet and fry on either side until they become tender and golden brown. Remove from heat and enjoy with fresh basil.

Calorie Estimate: 100

13. Black Bean Fiesta Salad

Ingredients

¼ Cup of Corn 4

Oz. of Lean Ground Turkey

2 Cups of Shredded Romaine Lettuce

5 Tortilla Chips, crumbled

½ Cup of Diced Tomatoes

¼ Cup of Black Beans, drained

1 Tbs. of Cotija Cheese

Directions

1. Start by browning the ground turkey in a skillet over medium heat. Stir in seasonings to enhance the flavor of the taco salad.

2. Remove the turkey from the pan and transfer to a bowl. Simply toss the rest of the ingredients together into the bowl and enjoy!

Calorie Estimate: 380

14. Authentic Garbanzo Salad

<u>Ingredients</u>

- 1 ½ Cups of Chopped Fennel Bulb
- 2 Garlic Cloves, minced
- 1 Cup of Tomato, chopped
- ¾ Cup of Red Onion, finely chopped
- ½ Tbs. of Extra Virgin Olive Oil
- 1 Oz. of Crumbled Feta Cheese
- ½ Cup of Fresh Basil Leaves, chopped
- 1 15 Oz. Can of Chickpeas, drained and rinsed
- 2 ½ Tbs. of Balsamic Vinegar

<u>Directions</u>

1. Simply combine all of the ingredients into a medium bowl and toss well. Let stand for approximately thirty minutes, then sprinkle the feta cheese over top. Enjoy!

Calorie Estimate: 140

15. Low Calorie White Bean Vegetable Dip

<u>Ingredients</u>

¼ Cup of a Can of White Beans, drained and rinsed

1 Tbs. of Chives, chopped

1 Tbs. of Fresh Lemon Juice

2 tsp. of Extra Virgin Olive Oil

1 ½ Cup of Assorted Fresh Vegetables (to dip)

Directions

1. Prepare your dip by combining the beans, lemon juice, olive oil, and chives in a small bowl. Do so by mashing the ingredients with a fork until a smooth consistency is achieved.
2. Serve your fresh vegetable dip with sliced bell peppers, cucumbers, carrots, cherry tomatoes, etc. Enjoy!

Calorie Estimate: 70

16. Classic Broccoli Salad

Ingredients

1 ½ Cup of Broccoli Florets

¼ Cup of Light Mayonnaise

2 Tbs. of Almonds, chopped

2 Tbs. of Chopped Red Onion

3 Slices of Cooked Bacon, chopped

½ Tbs. of Red Vinegar

Directions

1. In a medium bowl, combine together the broccoli, onion, bacon, and almonds.

2. In another bowl, mix together the vinegar and mayonnaise; and then season with salt and pepper.
3. Pour the fresh mayo dressing over the broccoli mixture and stir the contents until the vegetables are evenly coated.
4. Cover and place in the refrigerator for at least one hour before eating.

Calorie Estimate: 95

17. Chicken Salad

Ingredients

½ Cup of Shredded Chicken

1 Tbs. of Dijon Mustard

¼ of a Celery Stalk, cut into thin slices

½ Cup of Light Mayonnaise

½ of a Green Onion, chopped

2 Tbs. of Pecans, chopped

½ Tbs. of Dill, Minced

Directions

1. Start by combining the chicken, celery, and onion in a large bowl; tossing to thoroughly mix.
2. In a separate bowl, combine the remaining ingredients, using salt and pepper to enhance the flavor of the salad. Next, simply spoon the mayonnaise and mustard dressing over chicken and celery mix and stir the salad to incorporate all of the ingredients.

3. Place the bowl of chicken salad in the refrigerator and chill for at least two hours. Enjoy your salad with a side of whole-wheat crackers.

Calorie Estimate: 140

18. Zucchini Parmesan Pizza Boats

<u>Ingredients</u>

    2 Small Zucchinis

    1 tsp. of Extra Virgin Olive Oil

    1/3 Cup of Marinara Sauce

    ¼ Cup of Mini Pepperoni Slices

    1 tsp. of Minced Garlic

    1 Oz. of Grated Parmesan Cheese

    4 Oz. of Shredded Light Mozzarella Cheese

<u>Directions</u>

1. Begin your recipe by first preheating your oven to 400 degrees and preparing a baking sheet with parchment paper.

2. Now, cut the zucchinis into halves lengthwise and pat the inside of each half with a paper towel. Place the zucchinis on the baking sheet and set aside.

3. In a small bowl, combine the extra virgin olive oil and garlic. Then, use a spoon or brush to lightly coat the tops of the zucchini with the mixture. Next, season the vegetables with salt and pepper before layering your desired amount of marinara sauce over the zucchini halves.

4. Top the zucchini with mozzarella cheese and parmesan cheese. Then, layer the pepperoni slices on top to finish.

5. Place the baking sheet into the oven and cook for approximately twelve to fifteen minutes. Remove the vegetables from the oven and garnish with a sprinkle of fresh oregano.

Calorie Estimate: 112

19. Simple Organic Apple Chicken Salad

<u>Ingredients</u>

½ Tbs. of Olive Oil

1 Cup of Apple Chips

1 Boneless, Skinless Organic Chicken Breast

½ Cup of Pecans

5 Oz. of Mixed Greens

½ Cup of Diced Tomatoes

¼ of a Red Onion, Sliced Thin

¼ Cup of Gorgonzola Cheese, crumbled

<u>Ingredients for Homemade Dressing</u>

2 Tbs. of White Balsamic Vinegar

1 Pinch of Salt

1 Pinch of Pepper

½ Tbs. of Minced Garlic

6 Tbs. of Extra Virgin Olive Oil

Directions

1. Begin your recipe by first preheating your oven to 350 degrees and preparing a baking sheet with aluminum foil and cooking spray.

2. Next, lightly coat the chicken breast with olive oil, and use salt and pepper to season. Place the chicken onto the baking sheet and cook in the oven for approximately twenty minutes, or until the juices run clear.

3. Remove the chicken from the oven and let cool for at least five minutes. Then, shred the chicken breast with a fork.

4. In a medium bowl, toss together the remaining salad ingredients. In a separate bowl, simply combine your homemade vinaigrette dressing ingredients with a fork.

5. Add the chicken into the salad bowl, and top with the delicious dressing. Enjoy!

Calorie Estimate: 110

20. Crayfish and Horseradish Cocktail

Ingredients

1 Tbs. of Crème Fraiche

Juice of 1 Lime

1 Avocado

½ tsp. of Cream Horseradish Sauce

140g Package of Crayfish Tails

1 Chicory Head

Directions

1. Start by making the horseradish cream by simply mixing together the horseradish sauce, half of the lime juice, and the crème fraiche. Cover the sauce and set aside to chill in the refrigerator until it is needed.

2. Next, place one to two chicory leaves into a serving dish or on a large plate. Finely shred the remaining chicory to use as a garnish on the plate.

3. Now, slice the avocado, remove the pit, and peel off the outer skin. Thinly slice the avocado and place it onto the shredded chicory. Use the remaining lime juice to enhance the flavor.

4. Simply lay the crayfish tails on top of the plate and serve with the horseradish cream. Enjoy!

Chapter 3: Dinner for One: 20 Recipes to Cook at Home

1. Maple Salmon and Greens

<u>Ingredients</u>

    1 Tbs. of Maple Syrup

    ½ Tbs. of Chopped Shallot, finely chopped

    ½ Tbs. of Balsamic Vinegar

    1 Tbs. of Extra Virgin Olive Oil

    ½ Tbs. of Fresh Lemon Juice

    ¼ Cup of Shelled Edamame, cooked

    ½ Tbs. of Dijon Mustard

    1 tsp. of Fresh Rosemary

    2 5Oz. Fresh Skinless Salmon Fillets

    3 Oz. of Fresh Baby Spinach

    1 Tbs. of Chopped Toasted Walnuts

<u>Directions</u>

1. Start by combining the maple syrup, lemon juice, mustard, vinegar, and shallot in a saucepan. Season with salt and pepper to enhance the dish's flavor.

2. Take two tablespoons of the maple syrup and vinegar mixture and combine it in a separate bowl with the olive oil. Set this bowl aside to use as a dressing later.

3. Now, heat the remainder of the maple syrup and vinegar mixture over medium- high heat. Heat the glaze until it begins to boil, then reduce heat and let simmer for approximately five minutes. Do not cover the glaze.

4. Remove the saucepan from heat and stir in the rosemary snippets.

5. Next, preheat your broiler. Lay your fish filets over the unheated rack of the broiler pan. Brush the salmon filets with half of the glaze, then broil for approximately five minutes, placed six inches away from the heat.

6. After the first five minutes, flip the fish filets over and brush the side facing up with the remaining glaze. Continue broiling for another three to five minutes.

7. While your salmon is cooking, begin preparing your vegetables. Simply combine the edamame, spinach, nuts, salt, and pepper in a bowl. Toss the vegetables with the dressing to fully coat the salad.

8. Spoon your salad onto a plate and lay your salmon fillets on top. Enjoy!

Calorie Estimate: 450

2. Pasta with Ricotta, Served with Vegetables

Ingredients

    2 Oz. of Dried Whole Grain Penne Pasta

    ¾ Cup of Asparagus, cut into 1- in. pieces

    1 Tbs. of Fresh Basil

    ¾ Cup of Broccoli Florets

    ¼ Cup of Light Ricotta Cheese

1 tsp. of Dried Thyme, crushed

1 tsp. of Balsamic Vinegar

3 tsp. of Grated Parmesan Cheese

1 ½ tsp. of Extra Virgin Olive Oil

½ tsp. of Minced Garlic

½ Large Tomato, diced

<u>Directions</u>

1. Prepare and cook the penne pasta according to the instructions provided on the packaging. Do not add salt to the boiling water.
2. During the last three minutes that the pasta is cooking, add in the broccoli florets and asparagus. When the pasta is finished cooking, drain the water from the pot.
3. In a medium serving bowl, combine the herbs, olive oil, ricotta cheese, and garlic. Season with a dash of salt and pepper as well.
4. Next, add the cooked pasta and vegetables into the ricotta and herb mixture. Add in the diced tomato and toss together the ingredients until they are well combined.
5. Sprinkle the parmesan cheese onto the pasta and enjoy!

Calorie Estimate: 350

3. Black Bean Cakes and Guacamole

<u>Ingredients</u>

½ an Avocado, peeled with the pit removed

1 Tbs. of Fresh Cilantro

8 Oz. Can of Black Beans, drained and rinsed.

2 tsp. of Lime Juice

1 Slice of Whole Grain Bread, torn

½ Clove of Garlic

½ tsp. of Adobo Sauce

1 Egg, beaten

½ Plum Tomato, diced

Directions

1. To make the guacamole, start with mashing the avocado in a small bowl. Next, stir in the lime juice and season with salt and pepper. Cover the fresh guacamole and store in the refrigerator until you are ready to eat.

2. Now, put the torn bread into a food processor and pulse until the slice breaks down into coarse crumbs. Pour the crumbs into a separate bowl and put to the side for later.

3. Next, place the garlic and cilantro into the processor and pulse until the ingredients are finely chopped. Then, add in the beans, adobo sauce, and season with cumin. Continue processing until the beans are coarsely chopped and the ingredients pull away from the side of the container.

4. Now, spoon the mixture into the bread crumbs. Add in the beaten egg, and combine until the ingredients are well incorporated. Next, shape the black bean mixture into one or two ½ in.- thick patties.

5. Heat your grill to medium- high heat and lightly grease the rack of the grill pan. Place the patties onto the heated rack and cook for eight to ten minutes. Turn the patties once halfway through cooking.

6. Serve the black bean patties with the guacamole and tomato. Enjoy!

Calorie Estimate: 170

4. Thai- Inspired Chicken Wraps

<u>Ingredients</u>

    3 Oz. of Skinless, Boneless Chicken Breasts, cut into strips

    ½ Cup of Packaged Broccoli Slaw

    ¾ Tbs. of Peanut Butter

    1 ½ tsp. of Low Sodium Soy Sauce

    1 10- in. Whole Wheat Tortilla, warmed

    1 Tbs. of Water

    A Pinch of Ground Ginger

    A Dash of Minced Garlic

    A Pinch of Garlic Salt

<u>Directions</u>

1. Season the chicken strips with black pepper and the garlic salt. Next, prepare a skillet with cooking spray over medium- high heat.

2. Place the chicken in the skillet and cook for three minutes. Then, remove from the pan and keep warm in the microwave or oven.

3. Now, add the broccoli into the pan with a pinch of ground ginger. Cook the contents of the pan for three minutes, until the broccoli is crisp but tender. Remove the vegetables from the pan and set aside.

4. In a sauce pan set to low heat, combine the peanut butter, soy sauce, minced garlic, ginger, and water. Constantly which the ingredients until a smooth sauce forms.

5. Now, being assembling the wrap by first spreading the peanut sauce over the tortilla. Now, layer on the chicken strips and vegetables. Simply roll the tortilla to create the wrap and enjoy!

Calorie Estimate: 180

5. Greek- Inspired Quinoa

<u>Ingredients</u>

¼ Cup of Quinoa, uncooked

1 Plum Tomato, finely diced and seeded

½ Cup of Water

1 Tbs. of Extra Virgin Olive Oil

¼ Cup of Fresh Spinach, shredded

1 Tbs. of Fresh Lemon Juice

2 Tbs. of Chopped Red Onion

2 Tbs. of Feta Cheese, crumbled

1 Avocado, peeled, pitted, and thinly sliced

<u>Directions</u>

1. Start by bringing the quinoa to a boil in a small saucepan with water. Once the quinoa is boiling, reduce the heat, cover and let simmer for approximately fifteen minutes or until the water has been absorbed.

2. In a mixing bowl, stir together the quinoa, onion, tomato, and spinach. In a separate bowl, whisk the olive oil and lemon juice with a dash of salt.

3. Now, mix the lemon juice and oil dressing with the quinoa mixture.

4. Now, lay the spinach onto a plate. Top with the quinoa and garnish the avocado. Sprinkle the feta cheese over top and enjoy!

Calorie Estimate: 320

6. Mexican- Inspired Burrito Bowl

<u>Ingredients</u>

    3 oz. of Black Beans

    1 tsp. of Chicken Broth

    2 Tbs. of Non- Fat Greek Yogurt

    3 Tbs. of Red Cabbage, sliced thin

    3 Oz. of Cooked Grilled Chicken Breast, sliced thin

    2 Tbs. of Chunky Salsa

    A Pinch of Cayenne

    A Pinch of Cumin

    A Pinch of Garlic Powder

<u>Directions</u>

1. Start by microwaving the black beans with the chicken broth and spices on high heat for forty seconds.

2. Now, add the red cabbage into a medium bowl and top with the black bean mixture. Next, layer on the sliced chicken, salsa, and yogurt. Enjoy!

Calorie Estimate: 340

7. Low- Carb Cauliflower Lasagna

Note: This recipe will make three servings

Ingredients

    ¾ lb. of Cauliflower

    4 Oz. of Ricotta Cheese

    1 Tbs. of Extra Virgin Olive Oil

    1 tsp. of Red Pepper Flakes

    4 Oz. of No- Boil Lasagna Noodles

    1 Tbs. of Chicken Stock

    1 ½ Cup of Marinara Sauce

    ½ Cup of Grated Parmesan

Directions

1. Begin this recipe by preheating your oven to 450 degrees and preparing a baking sheet with parchment paper.
2. Now, cut your cauliflower into slices that are 1/3- in. thick. Allow the florets on the edges to fall off.
3. Toss all of your cauliflower pieces with the olive oil in a bowl, so that the vegetable is lightly coated with the oil. Then, evenly place the cauliflower onto the baking sheet and roast in the oven for approximately fifteen minutes.

4. Be sure to stir and flip the larger pieces of cauliflower halfway through the cooking time. Check to see if the florets are tender by poking them with a knife. Remove the vegetables from the oven and lightly season with the red pepper flakes.

5. Set the cauliflower aside and reduce the oven to 350 degrees.

6. In a small bowl, blend together the ricotta cheese, cinnamon, and chicken stock. Season with salt and pepper, then side aside.

7. Prepare a square baking dish with a layer or olive oil or cooking spray. Then, spread a spoonful of the tomato sauce on the bottom of the dish. Then, begin layering your lasagna, starting with the noodles.

8. Next, add a layer of the ricotta cheese mixture, then a third layer of the cauliflower. Next, add on another spoonful of tomato sauce, then parmesan cheese. Repeat the layers as many times as necessary until you have used all of your ingredients. The top layer should be the last of the noodles and parmesan cheese.

9. Now, securely cover your baking dish with aluminum foil and place your lasagna in the oven. Bake for forty minutes until the noodles are tender.

10. Uncover the dish and bake another few minutes so that the cheese on top browns. Then, remove from heat and let your lasagna sit for at least five minutes before eating it.

Calorie Estimate: 310

8. Classic Low- Carb Stuffed Peppers

Ingredients

2 Red Bell Peppers, halved and deseeded

½ White Onion, diced

3 Cloves of Garlic, chopped

¼ Cup of Diced Tomatoes

1 lb. of Ground Turkey Meat

2 Basil Leaves, chopped

1 Tbs. of Unrefined Coconut Oil

Directions

1. Preheat your oven to 375 degrees and prepare a roasting dish with cooking spray.
2. Place the red bell pepper halves into the roasting dish, facing down. Place I the oven for ten minutes.
3. While the red peppers are cooking, heat up the coconut oil in a large skillet over medium- high heat. Now, put the onions into the skillet and season with salt and pepper. Continue sautéing the onions until they become translucent and slightly brown.
4. Next, add in the tomatoes and garlic. Let the vegetables simmer for two minutes. Then, add in the meat and continue cooking the mixture until the turkey is done. Season with basil for added flavor.
5. Remove the red peppers from the oven and flip them over onto a plate. Carefully spoon the turkey stuffing into the pepper halves. Enjoy!

Calorie Estimate: 280

9. Low- Carb Sweet Potato Burger

Ingredients

- 1 Sweet Potato
- 1 Cup of Canned Chickpeas, drained and rinsed
- 2 Tbs. of Dry Quinoa
- 2 Tbs. of Whole Wheat Flour
- 1 Tbs. of Parsley
- 2 Tbs. of Extra Virgin Olive Oil
- 2 Tbs. of Dry Barley
- 1 ½ Red Bell Peppers

Directions

1. Preheat your oven to 390 degrees and bake your sweet potato for approximately forty- five minutes, until it becomes soft.
2. While the sweet potato bakes, cook your quinoa according to the packaging instructions. In a separate pot, cook the barely for approximately forty to fifty minutes.
3. Now, remove the stems and seeds from the red bell pepper and cut them into quarters. Also cut the half pepper in half as well. Roast the peppers for approximately twenty minutes.
4. When the sweet potato is done cooking and has cooled, combine it in the food processor with the beans, parsley, flour, pepper, and one tablespoon oil. Season with cumin, salt, and pepper.
5. Let the quinoa cool as you mix the beans with the quinoa and barely in another bowl.

6. Heat the remaining oil in a skillet over medium heat. Place large spoonfuls of the entire mixture into the skillet and use the back of a spoon to pat the mixture flat. This is the technique you will need to use to form 'burger' patties. Brown either side of the patties then remove from heat.

7. Serve your burger patties on a bun and enjoy!

Calorie Estimate: 200

10. Filling Sweet Potato Salad

<u>Ingredients</u>

2 Sweet Potatoes

2 Oz. of Extra Virgin Olive Oil

¼ Cup of Sliced Spring Onions

1 Tbs. of Fresh Mint Leaves, minced

4 Tbs. of Red Wine Vinegar

1 Red Bell Pepper, seeded, cored, and cut into quarters

1 Tbs. of Orange Zest

1 ½ Oz. of Raisins

2 tsp. of Ground Cumin

1 Chili, minced

<u>Directions</u>

1. Begin cooking this recipe by preheating your oven to 390 degrees. As your oven is heating up, peel your sweet potatoes and cut them into small cubes. Then, place the bite-size cubes onto a baking sheet lined with cooking spray.

2. Next, drizzle half of the olive oil over top of the potatoes and season with salt and pepper. Place the baking sheet into the oven for thirty minutes, until the cubes become tender.

3. While the potatoes cook, start preparing the dressing. Simply blend the remaining olive oil with the bell pepper, vinegar, orange sext, and cumin. Puree the ingredients until smooth.

4. Remove the potatoes from the oven and toss them in with the spring onions, chili, mind, and raisins. Add in at least three tablespoons of your homemade dressing, tossing to fully cover the potatoes. Season with salt and pepper and enjoy!

Calorie Estimate: 260

11. Easy Roast Beef Specialty

*Note: This recipe will make more than one serving. *

Ingredients

    1 lb. of Boneless Beef Rib Roast, warmed to room temperature

    ¼ Cup of Light Sour Cream

    ½ Tbs. of Mixed- Color Peppercorns

    1 ½ Tbs. of Horseradish

Directions

1. Start by heating your oven to 375 degrees and prepare a heavy cooking pan with cooking spray.

2. Pour the peppercorns into a plastic Ziploc bag, and crush them with the bottom of the pan.

3. Put the beef into the roasting pan and season with the peppercorn and a dash of salt. Carefully press the peppercorns into the roast so that they adhere to the meat.

4. Place the roast beef into the oven and cook for approximately ninety minutes. When it is done cooking, transfer the roast into a cutting board and loosely cover with aluminum foil. Let the roast rest for at least ten minutes before cutting.

5. As the roast is cooking, begin preparing the sauce. In a small bowl, mix together the horseradish, sour cream, and a dash of salt and pepper. Serve this dressing with the roast beef and enjoy!

Calorie Estimate: 400

12. Chicken Milanese Served with a Green Salad

Ingredients

    1 Tbs. of Extra Virgin Olive Oil

    1 6 Oz. Boneless, Skinless Chicken Breast

    ¼ tsp. of Ground Coriander

    1 Tbs. of Fresh Lemon Juice

    2 ½ Oz. of Baby Arugula

    2 Radishes, sliced

    ¼ Red Onion, Sliced

Directions

1. Begin cooking this recipe by first heating your grill to high heat. When the grill is hot, coat the grill gate with a bit of extra olive oil.

2. Next, slice the chicken breast horizontally, without cutting the filet all the way through. Season your chicken with the coriander, as well as salt and pepper. Then, place the chicken on the grill and cook the meat all the way through; which will take approximately three minutes on each side.

3. In a small bowl, combine the lemon juice, olive oil, as well as salt and pepper. Add in the radishes, onion, and arugula: toss the ingredients so that the salad is fully coated with the dressing.

4. Serve the fresh salad over the delicious grilled chicken, and enjoy!

Calorie Estimate: 300

13. Lamb Chops Served with Vegetables

Ingredients

½ Tbs. of Extra Virgin Olive Oil

2 1 ½ -in. Thick Lamb Chops

2 Shallots, sliced in half

2 Plum Tomatoes, cut into quarters

2 Tbs. of Pitted Kalamata Olives

1 Tbs. of Fresh Parsley Leaves

Directions

1. Begin making this recipe by heating your oven to 400 degrees and prepare a large oven- proof skillet with extra olive oil. Place the skillet over medium- high heat.

2. Season your lamp with salt, pepper, and paprika. Place the lamb into the oven and cook for three minutes on each side.

3. Place the shallots into the skillet while the lamb is in the oven. Then, transfer the skillet and continue cooking the lamb and shallots for an additional five to seven minutes.

4. Remove the lamb from the oven and transfer onto a plate. Place the olives, tomatoes, and parsley into the skillet and toss together with the shallots.

5. Add the mixed vegetables onto the plate as a side and enjoy!

Calorie Estimate: 200

14. Savory Baby- Back Ribs

Ingredients

    2 Cloves of Garlic, chopped

    1 Rack of Baby- Back Ribs

    1 Tbs. of Brown Sugar

    ½ tsp. of Chili Powder

    ¼ tsp. of Cayenne Pepper

Directions

1. Use a small bowl to combine the brown sugar, cayenne, garlic, and chili powder. Add in a sprinkle of salt and pepper for enhanced flavor.

2. Rub your homemade seasoning onto the stack of ribs and let the meat sit for ten minutes.

3. While the ribs are resting, heat your grill to medium heat. Then, grill the ribs, covering the grill. Turn the meat occasionally until it is cooked through. This may take approximately twenty- five minutes.

Calorie Estimate: 600

15. Classic Savory Steak

Ingredients

¼ Cup of Parsley Leaves

½ Clove of Garlic, chopped

¼ Tbs. of Red Wine Vinegar

½ tsp. of Fresh Oregano

1 Tbs. of Extra Virgin Olive Oil

½ lb. of Skirt Steak

¼ Vidalia Onion, sliced into ¼- in. pieces

Directions

1. Finely chop the garlic, parsley, and oregano with a food processor. Then, transfer the mixture into a bowl, adding in the vinegar, oil, as well as salt and pepper. Mix the ingredients well.

2. Heat your broiler and cut the steaks into slightly smaller portions. Next, place the steak into a roasting pan and rub both sides of the fillets with the sauce.

3. Broil your steak slices for four minutes on each side to achieve a medium roast. Cover the roast with aluminum foil before placing into the oven. Remove the roast from the oven and let rest for five minutes before serving.

4. Serve your steak slices with the raw onions on top.

Calorie Estimate: 420

16. Low- Carb Coconut Shrimp

Ingredients

    2 Tbs. of Unsweetened Coconut Flakes

    1 ½ Tbs. of Whole Wheat Flour

    1 ½ Tbs. of Panko Breadcrumbs

    1 Egg White

    ¼ lb. of Large Shrimp, peeled and pat dry

Directions

1. Begin this recipe by preheating your oven to 450 degrees and preparing a backing sheet with cooking spray.

2. In a baking dish, combine together the coconut, whole wheat flour, and panko breadcrumbs.

3. In a small bowl, beat the egg white until it becomes frothy. Now, season the shrimp with salt and pepper. Then, toss the shrimp into the egg whites.

4. Remove the shrimp from the bowl of egg whites and allow the excess egg to drip off the meat. Lightly coat the shrimp in the crumb and coconut mixture; pressing the coating so that it adheres to the meat.

5. Lay the shrimp onto the baking sheet and lightly coat the shrimp with cooking spray. Place the baking sheet into the oven and bake for eight to ten minutes, until the shrimp become golden brown.

6. Remove from the oven and enjoy!

Calorie Estimate: 200

17. Cabbage Detox Salad

<u>Ingredients</u>

1 Cup of Mixed Purple and Green Cabbage, finely shredded

2 Tbs. of Red and Yellow Peppers, diced

1 Avocado, pit removed and thinly sliced

1 ½ Tbs. of Hemp Oil

½ Tbs. of Lime Juice

½ Oz. of Hemp Seeds

1 Tbs. of Chopped Cilantro

<u>Directions</u>

1. Simply combine the ingredients together in a large bowl. Use your hands to tenderize the cabbage and mash the avocado. Enjoy!

Calorie Estimate: 350

18. Classic Paleo Meatballs

*Note: This recipe will make more than one serving. *

Ingredients

- 1 Egg
- 2 Tbs. of Cilantro, finely chopped
- 1/3 Cup of Almond Meal
- 1 Tbs. of Ground Cumin
- 1 lb. of Lean Ground Beef
- 4 Tbs. of Unrefined Coconut Oil
- 1 tbs. of Ginger, minced
- 2 Tbs. of Tomato Paste
- 2 Tbs. of Chopped Parsley Leaves
- 1 ½ Cup of Diced Tomatoes
- ½ Onion, diced
- 2 Cloves of Garlic, chopped
- 1 tsp. of Red Pepper Flakes
- Zest of 1 Lemon
- ¾ Cup of Chicken Stock
- 2 Tbs. of Clarified Butter

Directions

1. In a large bowl, combine the tomato paste with the egg until you achieve a smooth consistency. Then, add in the garlic, cilantro, cumin, and ginger until the ingredients are well incorporated.

2. Now, add in both the almond meal and beef. Enhance the flavor of your meatballs with salt and pepper.

3. Next, create meatballs with the meat mixture. Use your hands to roll the balls into spheres that are approximately 1- in. round in diameter.

4. Heat a large skillet over medium high heat, and place the coconut oil into the pan. Place the meatballs in the skillet and cook until they are golden brown on all sides.

5. Set the meatballs aside and prepare the sauce. Heat the butter in a saucepan and sauté the onion and garlic in the pan for four minutes. Add in the lemon zest and continue cooking for an additional minute.

6. Next, add the chicken stock, tomatoes, and red pepper flakes into the sauce pan and simmer for approximately six minutes.

7. Transfer your meatballs onto a plate and serve with a generous serving of your homemade sauce. Enjoy!

Calorie Estimate: 350

19. Cauliflower Mac and Cheese Substitute

Ingredients

2 Tbs. of Butter

1 Tbs. of Coconut Flour

½ Onion, minced

7 Oz. of Light Coconut Milk

½ Clove of Garlic, minced

½ Large Head of Cauliflower, broken into small florets

¼ tsp. of Dry Mustard

¾ Cup of Shredded Extra- Sharp Cheddar Cheese

2 Tbs. of Grated Parmesan Cheese

1 Tbs. of Ground Flaxseed

Directions

1. Heat a saucepan over medium- high heat. Add in half of the butter to the saucepan and cook the onion until it becomes lightly browned. Next, add in the garlic and continue cooking for another minute or so.

2. Now, add the coconut flour into the saucepan and stir the mixture constantly for three minutes until the ingredients are lightly browned. Then, stir in the coconut milk and mustard and bring the mixture to a boil. Stir the contents constantly.

3. Remove the saucepan from heat and stir in the cheddar cheese and cauliflower until well blended. Next, spoon the cauliflower into a baking dish and set aside for now.

4. Now, combine the parmesan cheese, remaining butter, and flaxseeds. Now, sprinkle the cheese over top of the cauliflower casserole.

5. Place the serving dish into the oven and bake for approximately thirty minutes, until the cheese start bubbling. Enjoy!

Calorie Estimate: 370

20. Low Calorie Buffalo Wings

Ingredients

½ lb. of Chicken Drumettes and Wings

¼ Tbs. of Butter

1 Sprig of Fresh Thyme

¾ Cup of Hot Sauce

2 Cloves of Garlic, crushed

Directions

1. Start by preheating your oven to 375 Degrees, with the fan on. Coat a baking pan with cooking spray.

2. In a medium mixing bowl, season your chicken with salt and pepper.

3. Heat a skillet over low heat and allow your butter to melt. Add in the garlic and thyme and let simmer for three minutes. Add in the hot sauce, and continue stirring.

4. Pour the hot sauce mixture over the chicken, tossing the wings and drumettes so that the sauce fully coats the meat. Now, allow the chicken to marinate in the refrigerator for at least thirty minutes.

5. Once the chicken is done marinating, place the wings and drumettes into the baking dish and put into the oven. Bake the chicken for approximately thirty minutes. Flip the wings and baste them so that the meat cooks fully through.

6. Continue baking for another twenty-five minutes after flipping the wings. Then, remove the baking pan from the oven. Allow the wings to cool slightly before enjoying them with a side of blue cheese dip!

Calorie Estimate: 360

Chapter 4: 10 Sweet Desserts that Curb Cravings

1. Sweet Energizing Green Popsicles

Ingredients

1 Avocado

½ Cup of Almond Milk

1 Tbs. of Matcha Powder

½ Cup of Non- Fat Greek Yogurt

2 Tbs. of Organic Honey

2 Tbs. of Water

1 Tbs. of Vanilla Extract

Directions

1. Start by cutting your avocado in half lengthwise. Remove the pit from the avocado, then cut the fruit into cubes.
2. Blend the avocado cubes, almond milk, yogurt, and tablespoons of water.
3. When the mixture is blended so that it has a smooth consistency. Then, add in the matcha, vanilla, and honey and mix well.
4. Next, pour the avocado mixture into popsicle molds and allow to freeze overnight. To remove the popsicles from the molds, simply run the container under hot water. Enjoy!

Calorie Estimate: 210

2. Strawberry and Banana Cream Delight

<u>Ingredients</u>

    ½ of a Banana

    8 Strawberries

    4 Tbs. of Vanilla Greek Yogurt

    1 Tbs. of Sliced Almonds

<u>Directions</u>

1. Start by mashing the banana with a fork inside a small bowl. Next, mix the yogurt and banana together to create the filling.

2. Cut off the tops of the strawberries and gently scoop out the middle of the berries to create a bowl-shape in the fruit.

3. Next, fill each strawberry with the banana filling and top with the sliced almonds. Enjoy!

Calorie Estimate: 140

4. Homemade Frozen Strawberry Yogurt

<u>Ingredients</u>

    2 Cups of Frozen Strawberries

    1 ½ Tbs. of Organic Honey

    ¼ Cup of Non- Fat Yogurt

    ½ Tbs. of Lemon Juice

Directions

1. First pour the strawberries, honey, lemon juice, and yogurt into the food processor. Pulse the fruit in the processor until the you achieve a creamy consistency.

2. Immediately serve the frozen yogurt, or place the dessert into an airtight container and store in the freezer for later.

Calorie Estimate: 110

3. Low Calorie Coffee Chocolate Mouse

Ingredients

1 ¼ tsp. of Dry Gelatin

½ tsp. of Vanilla Extract

¼ Cup of Brewed Coffee, still hot

½ Cup of Heavy Whipping Cream

½ tsp. of Instant Espresso

1 Cup of Ricotta Cheese

1 tsp. of Vanilla Liquid Stevia

A Pinch of Salt

Directions

1. Start by pour the dry gelatin into the hot coffee and stir until the powder fully dissolves. Set the bowl aside and allow the liquid to cool slightly.

2. Next, place the ricotta cheese, vanilla, salt, espresso, and stevia into a standing mixer. Or use a hand mixer to combine the ingredients. Blend the contents together until well combined.

3. Now, pour the coffee mixture into the ricotta batter and blend until well incorporated. Next, add in the whipping cream and blend the batter on high speed until the mousse is fully thickened and whipped.

4. Place the dessert into the refrigerator for two hours. Enjoy!

Calorie Estimate: 165

4. Low- Carb Cheesecake Bites

Ingredients

The Crust:

½ Cup of Gingersnap Cookies

¾ Tbs. of Melted Coconut Oil

The Filling

4 Oz. of Cream Cheese, softened and at room temperature

1 ½ Tbs. of Agave Syrup

2 Tbs. of a Beaten Egg

½ tsp. of Vanilla Extract

½ tsp. of Lemon Juice

Directions

1. Preheat your oven to 350 degrees and prepare a mini cupcake tray with liners.

2. Start by making the crust. First, place the gingersnaps into a food processor and pulse the cookies until crumbs have formed. Then, pour the crumbs into a small bowl stir in the melted coconut oil.

3. Use a tablespoon to add the crumbs into each muffin mold and press the crust down to flatten it.

4. Now it is time to make the cheesecake portion of the dessert. Start by beating the cream cheese with the agave syrup until the batter is light and fluffy.

5. Next, add in the egg and continue beating the batter. Then, add the vanilla extract, a pinch of salt, and lemon juice into the batter. Beat the cream cheese mixture until you achieve a smooth consistency.

6. Spoon a tablespoon onto each mini mold until all the batter has been used. Place the tray into the oven and bake for fifteen minutes.

7. Remove the cakes from the oven and allow to cool on a wire rack for ten minutes. Once the cakes have cooled, place the tray into the refrigerator and enjoy whenever you like!

Calorie Estimate: 60

5. Simple Strawberry Cake

Ingredients

3 Tbs. of Whole Wheat Flour

4 tsp. of Honey

1 Tbs. of Strawberry Protein Powder

½ Tbs. of Coconut Oil

¼ tsp. of Baking Powder

2 tsp. of Vanilla Low- Fat Greek Yogurt

1 ½ Tbs. of Vanilla Almond Milk

A Pinch of Salt

Directions

1. In a medium bowl, combine the flour, strawberry powder, salt, and baking powder. Set the bowl aside.

2. Next, combine the honey and coconut oil in a microwave- safe bowl. Place the bowl in the microwave and heat for thirty seconds.

3. Now, create a well in the middle of the bowl of dry ingredients and pour the coconut oil mixture into the center. Also add in the yogurt and almond milk. Then, stir all of the ingredients together to create a smooth batter.

4. Coat the inside of a mug with cooking spray before pouring the batter into the cup. Then, microwave the batter for a minute and ten seconds. Watch your cake closely to make sure that it does not grow too big and splatter.

5. Let the cake cool for one minute before enjoying with a serving of sweet strawberries!

Calorie Estimate: 110

6. Indulgent Chocolate Mug Cake

Ingredients

1 Tbs. of Whole Wheat Flour

1 Tbs. of Unsweetened Cocoa Powder

1 Tbs. of Low Fat Vanilla Yogurt

1 Tbs. of Sugar

A Pinch of Baking Soda

A Pinch of Salt

Directions

1. Simply combine all of the ingredients in a large mug. Then, just place the mug into the microwave and cook for one minute and ten seconds. Enjoy!

Calorie Estimate: 100

7. Festive Apple Cinnamon Dessert

Ingredient

1 Cup of Sliced Apple, peeled and cored

½ Tbs. of Cinnamon

1 tsp. of Brown Sugar

2 Tbs. of Water

½ Package of Instant Brown Sugar Cinnamon Quaker Oatmeal

Directions

1. Start by placing the apples into a baking dish. In a small bowl, combine the brown sugar and water. Then, carefully pour the mixture over the apple slices.

2. Toss the apples to coat them in the brown sugar. Next, sprinkle the apple slices with cinnamon and the oatmeal.

3. Preheat your oven to 450 degrees. Place the baking dish into the oven and bake for fifteen minutes. Then, remove the tray from the oven and stir the contents.

4. Return the apples into the oven and continue cooking for another ten minutes. Serve the fruit immediately and enjoy!

Calorie Estimate: 90

8. Baked Grapefruit Dessert

<u>Ingredients</u>

    1 Grapefruit

    1 tsp. of Cinnamon

<u>Directions</u>

1. Start by preheating the oven to 400 degrees and prepare a baking sheet with cooking spray.
2. Slice the grapefruit in half. Use a knife to carefully loosen the segments without cutting through the grapefruit peel.
3. Next, place the halves onto the baking sheet and sprinkle the cinnamon over top of the fruit. Then, place the tray into the oven and bake for approximately twenty minutes.
4. Remove the fruit from the oven and let cool for at least five minutes before eating.

Calorie Estimate: 40

9. Sweet Protein Powered Peanut Butter Balls

<u>Ingredients</u>

    ½ Cup of Creamy Peanut Butter

    1 Cup of Powdered Sugar

3 Tbs. of Salted Butter, softened

Directions

1. Start by mixing the peanut butter with the butter in a bowl. Then, add in the powdered sugar and combine completely until the dough forms into a large ball.

2. Cover the peanut butter dough and allow to sit for approximately fifteen minutes or place into the refrigerator so that the dough becomes firm.

3. Next, shape the peanut butter into 1-in. thick balls and place them onto a baking sheep. Place into the refrigerator to chill and enjoy!

Calorie Estimate: 60

10. Energizing Oatmeal Balls

Ingredients

¾ Cup of Rolled Oats

¼ Cup of Vanilla Weigh Protein Powder

¼ tsp. of Cinnamon

½ Tbs. of Chia Seeds

¼ Cup of Creamy Peanut Butter

1 ½ Tbs. of Honey

½ tsp. of Vanilla Extract

3 Tbs. of Dark Chocolate Chips

1 Tbs. of Almond Milk

Directions

1. In a large bowl, combine the oats, cinnamon, protein powder, and chia seeds.

2. Next, add in the peanut butter, vanilla, and honey. Stir together until the ingredients are well incorporated. Add in the chocolate chips and milk by using your hands.

3. Take the oatmeal into your hands and roll into small balls and place into a container. Place the oatmeal balls into the refrigerator for thirty minutes and enjoy!

Calorie Estimate: 40

Chapter 5: 10 Crockpot Single and Double Serving Recipes

1. Spicy Vegetables

<u>Ingredients</u>

- ¾ Cup of Vegetable Broth
- 5 Oz. of Canned Diced Tomatoes
- 5 Oz. of Refried Beans
- ½ Onion, chopped
- 1 Clove of Garlic, minced
- ¼ tsp. of Cumin
- 1 tsp. of Paprika
- 5 Oz. of Black Beans, cooked
- ½ Cup of Frozen Kernels
- ¼ Cup of Western- Style Vegetables
- 1 tsp. of Hot Sauce
- ¼ tsp. of Oregano

<u>Directions</u>

1. In place of a crockpot, use a large non- stick pot instead. Prepare the pot with cooking spray and sauté the onion until it browns. Then, add in the garlic and continue cooking for another minute.

2. Add in the rest of the ingredients and stir. Allow the chili to cook for thirty minutes and enjoy with a side of tortilla chips!

Calorie Estimate: 190

2. Tomato Soup with Lentils

Ingredients

- 1 Tbs. of Extra Virgin Olive Oil
- 2 Oz. of Pancetta Cheese, chopped
- ¾ Cup of Brown Lentils, rinsed
- 1 Onion, finely chopped
- 1 Carrot, chopped
- 1 Stalk of Celery, diced
- 4 Cups of Water
- 2 Tbs. of Tomato Paste
- ½ Bay Leaf
- 1 Tbs. of Red Wine Vinegar

Directions

1. In a medium skillet, heat the olive oil over medium heat. Add the pancetta into the skillet and cook for five minutes.
2. Add the onion, water, celery, lentils, tomato paste, bay leaf, and carrot into the crockpot. Use a spatula to spoon the pancetta into the pot. Stir the ingredients to combine.

3. Cover the crockpot and cook on low heat for eight hours. Season with the vinegar, as well as salt and pepper. Enjoy!

Calorie Estimate: 150

3. Pulled BBQ Pork

Ingredients

2 Tbs. of Dark Rum

1 Yellow Onion, sliced

1 ¼ lb. Pork Tenderloin

Juice of ½ a Lemon

1 Cup of Barbeque Sauce

½ tsp. of Chili Powder

A Pinch of Garlic Powder

Directions

1. Start by combining the chili powder, garlic powder, as well as salt and pepper into a bowl. Next, drizzle the pork with the lemon juice, and then rub the spices onto the meat.
2. Place the tenderloin into a Ziploc bag and marinate the meat in the refrigerator for two hours.
3. Next, put the onion into the bottom of the slow cooker. Then, remove the tenderloin from the bag and slice the meat into 1- in. thick cubes. Put the cubes on top of the onions.
4. In a small bowl, combine the barbeque sauce and rum with a fork. Pour the sauce over top of the roast.

5. Cover the crockpot and cook on low heat for six hours. Then, shred the pork with a fork and enjoy!

Calorie Estimate: 180

4. Beef and Broccoli

<u>Ingredients</u>

½ lb. of Boneless Beef Chuck Roast, cut into thin slices

2 Tbs. of Dark Brown Sugar

1 Tbs. of Corn Starch

½ Cup of Beef Broth

½ Tbs. of Sesame Oil

1 Cup of Broccoli Florets

¼ cup of Low- Sodium Soy Sauce

¼ Cup of Brown Rice, cooked

1 Garlic Clove, minced

<u>Directions</u>

1. Whish the beef stock, brown sugar, garlic, soy sauce, and sesame oil in the crockpot bowl. Place the beef into the crockpot and gently toss to coat the meat.
2. Turn the crockpot on to low heat and cook the beef for six hours.
3. After the cooking time is up: in a small bowl, whisk together the cornstarch and two tablespoons of the liquid from the crockpot. Pour the mixture back into the crockpot and stir the contents.

4. Also add in the florets and cook on low for another thirty minutes. Serve the beef and broccoli over the rice and enjoy!

5. Spicy Taco Chili

<u>Ingredients</u>

    8 Oz. of Black Beans, rinsed and drained

    8 Oz. of Kidney Beans, rinsed and drained

    1 Clove of Minced Garlic

    ½ Onion, chopped

    ½ Jalapeno Pepper, minced

    ½ Green Bell Pepper, diced

    ¾ Cup of Frozen Corn

    1 Boneless, Skinless Chicken Breast

    4 Oz. of Tomato Sauce

    12 Oz. of Canned Diced Tomatoes, drained

    ½ Tbs. of Cumin

    ½ Tbs. of Chili Powder

    ½ tsp. of Oregano

<u>Directions</u>

1. Place all of the ingredients except for the chicken into the slow cooker. Stir everything together so that the mixture is well combined. Now, place the chicken on top of the mixture.

2. Cover the crockpot and cook on low heat for six hours. Stir the chicken occasionally. Thirty minutes before serving the dish, shred the chicken with two forks.

3. Enjoy the chili with a slice of low calorie corn bread or tortilla chips.

6. Fisherman's Stew

<u>Ingredients</u>

¼ lb. of Medium Shrimp, peeled and deveined

1 tsp. of Sugar

1 Cup of Quartered Tomatoes, sliced

½ Cup of Green Pepper, chopped

½ tsp. Fennel Seed

1 Tbs. of Extra Virgin Olive Oil

½ Cup of Leek, sliced

½ lb. of Cod, cut into 1-in. cubes

1 Clove of Garlic, chopped

½ Cup of Baby Carrots, sliced

1 Bay Leaf

1 Cup of Water

4 Oz. of Clam Juice

<u>Directions</u>

1. Combine the olive oil, garlic, and leek in the slow cooker and mix together well. Next, pour in the carrots,

fennel seed, tomatoes, clam juice, and bay leaf. Stir the contents of the slow cooker to combine.

2. Cover the slow cooker and set to low heat setting for eight hours.

3. Twenty minutes before serving, add in the remaining ingredients and continue cooking.

Calorie Estimate: 180

7. Homemade Apple Oatmeal

Ingredients

1 ½ Gala Apples, cored and diced

1 Cup of Steel Cut Oats

1 Cup of Milk

2 Cups of Water

1 tsp. of Vanilla Extract

1 tsp. of Cinnamon

Directions

1. Prepare the slow cooker with cooking spray and place the diced apples into the pot. Then, add in the steel cut oats, water, milk, cinnamon, and vanilla extract.

2. Turn your slow cooker on to low heat, cover, and cook the oatmeal for seven hours.

3. Stir the contents and enjoy! You can store any leftover oatmeal for up to a week.

Calorie Estimate: 180

8. Simple Egg Breakfast

<u>Ingredients</u>

    2 Slices of Bacon

    2 Oz. of Fresh Mushrooms

    ¾ Tbs. of Butter

    4 Eggs

    1 Large Tomato, quartered and sliced

    ¼ Cup of Milk

    ½ Cup of Shredded Cheddar Cheese

    A Pinch of Salt

    A Pinch of Pepper

    2 Oz. of Condensed Cream of Mushroom Soup

    ½ Tbs. of Chives

<u>Directions</u>

1. Use a skillet to cook the bacon until crispy, reserving a tablespoon of the melted fat for later. Add the mushrooms into the skillet with the remaining bacon fat and cook them until tender. Then, remove the mushrooms from the skillet and set aside.

2. Clean the skillet with a paper towel. Now, melt the butter in the skillet over medium heat. In a small bowl, beat the eggs, adding in the half and half as well as the salt and pepper for seasoning.

3. Place the egg mixture into the skillet and cook until the eggs are firm but moist. Stir in the soup and chives.

4. Pour the eggs into the crockpot and layer the remaining ingredients on top. Keep on warm setting for up to three hours and enjoy whenever you like!

Calorie Estimate: 290

9. Easy Baked Potato Recipe

Ingredients

2 Baked Potatoes (or however many you want)

Aluminum Foil

Directions

1. Start by stabbing the potatoes with a fork. Then, wrap the potatoes in the foil and place them into the crockpot.
2. Cover the pot and cook on high heat for approximately three hours.

Calorie Estimate: 120

10. Spinach and Artichoke Dip

Ingredients

4 Oz. of Frozen Spinach, thawed and squeezed

¼ tsp. of Garlic Salt

4 Oz. of Artichoke Hearts, quartered, drained, and chopped

½ Cup of Shredded Swiss Cheese

¼ Cup of Alfredo Pasta Sauce

¼ Cup of Mayonnaise

1 Handful of Pita Chips or Bread to Dip

<u>Directions</u>

1. Mix all of the ingredients in the slow cooker, excluding the bread or chips.
2. Cover your crockpot and set it to low heat setting. Cook your dip for three to four hours, then enjoy!

Calorie Estimate: 130

Chapter 6: 25 Meal Replacement Smoothies

1. Protein Power- Up

<u>Ingredients</u>

>1 Cup of Ice Cubes

>¾ Cup of Almond Milk

>1 Frozen Banana

>¼ Cup of Hemp Granola

>1 Scoop of Vanilla Whey Protein Powder

<u>Directions</u>

>Simply combine all of the ingredients in a blender until you achieve a smooth consistency.

Calorie Estimate: 430

2. Green Banana Smoothie

<u>Ingredients</u>

>1 Frozen Banana

>½ Cup of Baby Spinach

>1 ½ Tbs. of Creamy Peanut Butter

>1 Cup of Almond or Soy Milk

<u>Directions</u>

Simply combine all of the ingredients in a blender until you achieve a smooth consistency.

Calorie Estimate: 320

3. Tempting Chocolate Peanut Butter Blend

<u>Ingredients</u>

    1 Frozen Banana

    ½ Cup of Vanilla Almond Milk

    2 Tbs. of Creamy Peanut Butter

    1 Cup of Ice

    ½ Tbs. of Honey

    ¾ Tbs. of Cocoa Powder

<u>Directions</u>

Simply combine all of the ingredients in a blender until you achieve a smooth consistency.

Calorie Estimate: 350

4. Berry Green Smoothie

<u>Ingredients</u>

    1 Cup of Blueberries

    1 Cup of Kale Leaves, stems removed

    2 Tbs. of Rolled Oats

    1 Cup of Soy Milk

    ½ of a Banana

1 ½ Tbs. of Almond Butter

Directions

Simply combine all of the ingredients in a blender until you achieve a smooth consistency.

Calorie Estimate: 300

5. Apple Cinnamon Dessert Smoothie

Ingredients

8 Oz. of Coconut Water

1 Cup of Chopped Apple

5 Almonds

1 tsp. of Cinnamon

1 tsp. of Vanilla Extract

½ Scoop of Protein Powder, unsweetened

1 Tbs. of Ground Flaxseed

Directions

Simply combine all of the ingredients in a blender until you achieve a smooth consistency.

Calorie Estimate: 230

6. Sweet Carrot Smoothie

Ingredients

½ Cup of Carrot Juice

¾ Cup of Vanilla Almond Milk

5 Ice Cubes

1 Frozen Banana

1 Scoop of Vanilla Whey Protein Powder

¼ tsp. of Ground Cinnamon

Directions

Simply combine all of the ingredients in a blender until you achieve a smooth consistency.

7. Morning Breakfast Smoothie

Ingredients

3 Oz. of Coconut Water

½ Tbs. of Organic Honey

¼ Cup of Low- Fat Cottage Cheese

½ Frozen Banana

1 Cup of Ice Cubes

½ Tbs. of Chia Seeds

1 Cup of Kale Leave, stems removed

½ Cup of Pineapple Chunks

Directions

Simply combine all of the ingredients in a blender until you achieve a smooth consistency.

Calorie Estimate: 370

8. Classic Mango Smoothie

Ingredients

- ¼ Cup of Mango, cut into cubes
- ½ Cup of Fat- Free Vanilla Yogurt
- ¼ Cup of Mashed Avocado
- 1 Tbs. of Lime Juice
- ½ Cup of Mango Juice
- ½ Tbs. of Sugar
- 2 Scoops of Whey Protein Powder
- 6 Ice Cubes

Directions

Simply combine all of the ingredients in a blender until you achieve a smooth consistency.

Calorie Estimate: 300

9. Blueberry Soothing Smoothie

Ingredients

- 1 Cup of Skim Milk, chilled
- 1 Cup of Frozen Blueberries
- 1 Tbs. of Flaxseed Oil, cold- pressed

Directions

Simply combine all of the ingredients in a blender until you achieve a smooth consistency.

Calorie Estimate: 270

10. Vanilla and Blueberry Smoothie

Ingredients

    1 Cup of Vanilla Soy Milk

    6 Oz. of Low Fat Vanilla Yogurt

    1 Cup of Blueberries

    1 Tbs. of Coconut Oil

    5 Ice Cubes

Directions

    Simply combine all of the ingredients in a blender until you achieve a smooth consistency.

Calorie Estimate: 440

11. Chocolate Raspberry Dessert

Ingredients

    ½ Cup of Almond Milk

    6 Oz. of Low- Fat Vanilla Yogurt

    4 Ice Cubes

    ¼ Cup of Dark Chocolate Chips

    1 Cup of Fresh Raspberries

Directions

    Simply combine all of the ingredients in a blender until you achieve a smooth consistency.

Calorie Estimate: 460

12. Peachy Keen Smoothie

Ingredients

- 1 Cup of Soy Milk
- 1 Cup of Frozen Peaches
- 1 tsp. of Coconut Oil

Directions

Simply combine all of the ingredients in a blender until you achieve a smooth consistency.

Calorie Estimate: 215

13. Citrus Morning Smoothie

Ingredients

- 1 Cup of Soy Milk
- 1 Tbs. of Coconut Oil
- 1 Orange, peeled and sliced into sections
- 6 Oz. of Lemon- Flavored Yogurt
- 4 Ice Cubes

Directions

Simply combine all of the ingredients in a blender until you achieve a smooth consistency.

Calorie Estimate: 420

14. Sweet Apple Smoothie

Ingredients

½ Cup of Soy Milk

1 tsp. of Apple Pie Spice

6 Oz. of Vanilla Yogurt

2 Tbs. of Creamy Peanut Butter

1 Medium Apple, peeled and chopped

5 Ice Cubes

Directions

Simply combine all of the ingredients in a blender until you achieve a smooth consistency.

Calorie Estimate: 470

15. Classic Strawberry Smoothie

Ingredients

1 Cup of Almond Milk

1 Cup of Frozen Strawberries

1 tsp. of Unrefined Coconut Oil

Directions

Simply combine all of the ingredients in a blender until you achieve a smooth consistency.

Calorie Estimate: 215

16. Green Detox Smoothie

Ingredients

½ of a Pear

½ of a Cucumber

1 tsp. of Cilantro

¼ of an Avocado

½ in. of Ginger

1 Cup of Kale, stems removed

½ of a Lemon

½ Cup of Coconut Water

Directions

Simply combine all of the ingredients in a blender until you achieve a smooth consistency.

Calorie Estimate: 280

17. Probiotic Blend

Ingredients

1 Cup of Papaya

Juice from ½ a Lime

1 Cup of Coconut Yogurt

1 Tbs. of Organic Honey

Directions

Simply combine all of the ingredients in a blender until you achieve a smooth consistency.

Calorie Estimate: 330

18. Refreshing Green Smoothie

Ingredients

- 1 Cup of Romaine Lettuce
- 1 Large Cucumber, peeled
- ½ Cup of Broccoli Florets
- 3 Carrots
- 1 Celery Stalk
- 1 Cup of Kale, stems removed
- 1 Green Apple, cut into quarters
- 2 Tomatoes
- ½ Lemon, peeled and cut into quarters

Directions

Simply combine all of the ingredients in a blender until you achieve a smooth consistency.

Calorie Estimate: 270

19. Savory Vegetable Blend

Ingredients

- 2 Red Bell Peppers
- 2 Large Tomatoes
- 1 Cup of Watercress
- 1 Carrot
- 1 Clove of Garlic
- 2 Stalks of Celery

1 Cup of Spinach

½ Cup of Coconut Water

Directions

Simply combine all of the ingredients in a blender until you achieve a smooth consistency.

Calorie Estimate: 310

20. Blueberry Lemon Smoothie

Ingredients

1 Cup of Alkaline Water

1 Lemon

½ Cup of Blueberries

Directions

Simply combine all of the ingredients in a blender until you achieve a smooth consistency.

Calorie Estimate: 230

21. Strawberry Goji Blast

Ingredients

1 Frozen Banana

1 Cup of Coconut Kefir Water

3 Tbs. of Goji Berries

½ Cup of Frozen Strawberries

Directions

Simply combine all of the ingredients in a blender until you achieve a smooth consistency.

Calorie Estimate: 275

22. Cacao and Hemp Smoothie

Ingredients

　　2 Tbs. of Hemp Seeds

　　10 Oz. of Alkaline Water

　　4 Red Endive Leaves

　　1Tbs. of Cacao Powder

　　½ Cup of Dark Cherries

　　1 Packet of Stevia Sugar

Directions

Simply combine all of the ingredients in a blender until you achieve a smooth consistency.

Calorie Estimate: 320

23. Fat Burning Green Smoothie

Ingredients

　　1 Cup of Coconut Water

　　2 Stalks of Celery

　　½ Cup of Flat- Leaf Parsley

　　1 Green Apple, peeled and cut into quarters

　　½ Cup of Spinach

1 Tbs. of Blue- Green Algae

½ Cup of Cilantro

½ tsp. of Fresh Ginger

Directions

Simply combine all of the ingredients in a blender until you achieve a smooth consistency.

Calorie Estimate: 280

24. Banana Cream Dessert Smoothie

Ingredients

1 Frozen Banana

½ tsp. of Vanilla Extract

4 Ice Cubes

1 Cup of Low- Fat Greek Yogurt

½ Cup of Almond Milk

2 Tbs. of Organic Honey

½ Graham Cracker

Directions

Simply combine all of the ingredients in a blender until you achieve a smooth consistency. Crush graham crackers and sprinkle on top as a garnish.

Calorie Estimate: 260

25. Very Berry Blast

Ingredients

- ½ Cup of Almond Milk
- ½ Cup of Frozen Blueberries
- ½ Cup of Frozen Strawberries
- 2 Medjool Dates
- ½ Cup of Frozen Blackberries
- ¼ Cup of Frozen Raspberries

Directions

Simply combine all of the ingredients in a blender until you achieve a smooth consistency.

Calorie Estimate: 240

Conclusion

Thank you again for downloading this book!

I hope this book was able to teach you some amazing new recipes to try, as well as inspire you to get started right away on your weight loss journey!

The next step is to start trying out all of these delicious recipes so that you can achieve all of your health and fitness goals!

Finally, if you enjoyed this book, please take the time to share your thoughts and post a review on Amazon. It'd be greatly appreciated!

Thank you and good luck!

Everyone knows the struggle of losing weight. We all wish that we could lose weight while still enjoying all of the delicious foods that probably caused the weight gain in the first place. After all, one of life's biggest questions is "why does unhealthy food taste so good when it is so bad for us?" Nutrition and fitness experts have spent decades trying to come up with the best solutions for helping people lose weight with special foods, programs, and supplements to make it happen.

However, to lose weight, burn fat, and keep those pounds off, you don't have to look any further than your own kitchen! All you need to do to lose weight is eat fresh, organic ingredients and learn how to make delicious meals on your own. This book contains more than ONE HUNDRED recipes that are guaranteed to help you lose weight and establish healthy, sustainable eating habits.

With twenty breakfast and lunch recipes, your tummy will be full and satisfied all day! And no one like wasting food that is the result of following recipes that are designed to feed a family of four. That is why all of these meals, especially the dinner recipes, only account for a single serving; to save you time, money, and food. Losing weight can be easy, if you know what to cook and what foods nourish your body!

Made in the USA
Monee, IL
27 October 2025